APPLE CIDER VINEGAR BENEFITS

Natural Weight Loss, Glowing Health and Skin, Natural Cures, and Alkaline Healing with Apple Cider Vinegar

BY
DANA LEE

Copyright © 2017 By Dana Lee
All Rights Reserved.

PositiveImpact Books
7579 E. Main Street, Suite 600a
Scottsdale, AZ 85251
USA

The following Book is reproduced below with the goal of providing information that is as accurate and as reliable as possible. Regardless, purchasing this Book can be seen as consent to the fact that both the publisher and the author of this book are in no way experts on the topics discussed within, and that any recommendations or suggestions made herein are for entertainment purposes only. Professionals should be consulted as needed before undertaking any of the action endorsed herein.

This declaration is deemed fair and valid by both the American Bar Association and the Committee of Publishers Association and is legally binding throughout the United States.

Furthermore, the transmission, duplication or reproduction of any of the following work, including precise information, will be considered an illegal act, irrespective whether it is done electronically or in print. The legality extends to creating a secondary or tertiary copy of the work or a recorded copy and is only allowed with express written consent of the Publisher. All additional rights are reserved.

The information in the following pages is broadly considered to be a truthful and accurate account of facts, and as such any inattention, use or misuse of the information in question by the reader will render any resulting actions solely under their purview. There are no scenarios in which the publisher or the original author of this work can be in any fashion deemed liable for any hardship or damages that may befall them after undertaking information described herein.

Additionally, the information found on the following pages is intended for informational purposes only and should thus be considered, universal. As befitting its nature, the information presented is without assurance regarding its continued validity or interim quality. Trademarks that mentioned are done without written consent and can in no way be considered an endorsement from the trademark holder.

"Twenty years from now you will be more disappointed by the things that you didn't do than by the ones you did do. So throw off the bowlines. Sail away from safe harbor. Catch the trade winds in your sails. Explore. Dream. Discover."

~ **Mark Twain**

Table of Contents

Introduction ....

Chapter 1: What is Apple Cider Vinegar? ....

    Regular vs. Raw Apple Cider Vinegar 8

    History and Overview of Apple Cider Vinegar 11

    Common Myths about Apple Cider Vinegar 16

Chapter 2: How to Make Raw Apple Cider Vinegar ....

    All about "The Mother" 26

    AMAZING Health Benefits of Apple Cider Vinegar 27

    Scientific Backed Claims of Apple Cider Vinegar 31

Chapter 3: Detoxing with Apple Cider Vinegar ....

    Natural Weight Loss using Apple Cider Vinegar 35

    Beauty Benefits of Apple Cider Vinegar 45

Chapter 4: Natural Cures with Apple Cider Vinegar ....

    Simple Apple Cider Recipes Anyone can do 54

    Natural Cures with Apple Cider Vinegar 64

    Recommended Apple Cider Vinegar Brands 67

    Where to Buy Apple Cider Vinegar 73

Chapter 5: Precautions and Recommendations ....

Chapter 6: Bonus: Apple Cider Vinegar in Treatment of Cellulite ....

Conclusion ....

INTRODUCTION

The goal of this book is to positively impact the Reader's experience in any way possible, even if just a minuscule amount, be it from a word, sentence, idea or comment in this book; then we have made a positive impact and achieved our goal.

"Apple Cider Vinegar – Is one of the most under-rated natural health supplements out there – WHY?"

I created this book because I am so sick of people being charged high prices for sophisticated health supplements, mostly which are not natural. Apple cider vinegar is available in most food stores and has huge life-changing effects on health and appearance. I speak from personal experience.

The science and history for apple cider vinegar's health benefits are tremendous and go back for thousands of years! Compare this fact to some of the modern health supplements being used.

My Quick Personal Story With Apple Cider Vinegar

When I was only 26 years old I was suffering from multiple symptoms of poor nutrition and stress.

- Weight issues

- Spiking blood pressure syndrome

- Weird sensations in my ankles and feet if standing for long periods

- Bad skin or appearance – generally always feeling unhealthy.

At that time I worked a government job on 3rd shift for over 6 years. I was not healthy at all and was borderline pre-diabetic; I weighed nearly 205 pounds, and was always feeling sick or tired.

After several 'wake-up calls" I eventually started a manageable work-out routine and ran 1-2 miles every other day, and that helped me a little, but my average blood pressure was around 160/90 and I still had a high body fat percentage. I wasn't over-weight but I still had a lot of subcutaneousfat, it was very strange and hard to figure out how to get rid of it.

When I reached the age of 29, I quit my job to become an entrepreneur and decided to do whatever it also took to reclaim my health since I was going to need it now. After a few more scares with super high blood pressure episodes and just generally always feeling sick, I discovered one of my first health supplements that would begin the health turnaround for me.

I must say, my personal experience with Apple Cider Vinegar for health benefits has been very noticeable, especially when I drink it consistently. All my biomarkers are very strong and I hover around 8-10% body fat. I do not eat any kind of special diet, just clean healthy food, and the apple cider vinegar in morning or before bed.

Although this was only ONE component of my new healthy lifestyle, it has played a major, if not the best, role in my drastic health and energy improvements. The truth is that I actually feel and look significantly better than I did when I was 29, and I wrote this at age 39.

This book is for someone just starting off in their quest for natural, healthy and beneficial supplementation; Apple Cider Vinegar is definitely something that has worked for a lot of people for a very long time. How can we ignore such a great history of positive results revolving around something so readily available in our stores and so affordable?

Apple cider vinegar has been called a superfluid, capable of doing everything from polishing your furniture to lowering your cholesterol levels. In this book, we will go over some of the anecdotal and scientific benefits of this fluid. Here is some of what apple cider vinegar can do:

Helps Reduce Appetite:

A study done in Sweden in 2005 discovered that people were more satisfied and fuller for longer periods when they ate bread along with vinegar, as opposed to by itself. The great ingredient in vinegar that reduces appetite is thought to be acetic acid.

This substance can help to lower foods' glycemic indexes. In other words, it slows down the rate that sugars get released into your blood stream, reducing your urge to eat more.

Lowers Fat Levels in the Body:

Many people insist that apple cider vinegar can help to shed weight, but there isn't as much scientific evidence for this. One study, done in Japan, however, showed that overweight people who drank acetic acid with water over about three months showed significant weight loss.

Lowers Levels of Bad Cholesterol:

A study done in 2012 by Life Science found that consuming apple cider vinegar over two months could reduce bad blood lipids significantly. These harmful blood lipids add to high levels of cholesterol.

Makes your Hair Shinier:

Apple cider vinegar can be used as a conditioner supplement or replacement. Just add one part apple cider vinegar to an equal amount of water and let it soak on your hair for a few minutes, then rinse thoroughly.

The rinsing step is important unless you want to smell like vinegar! These are just a few examples of what apple cider vinegar can do, but the rest of this book will go into detail about the other wonders this miracle liquid can offer you.

The final chapter will explore a bonus subject, using apple cider vinegar to cure and get rid of cellulite. We will also cover some other natural methods to use along with the vinegar for extra effectiveness in this.

Thank you for Choosing this Book:

There are plenty of books on this subject on the market, thanks again for choosing this one! Every effort was made to ensure it is full of as much useful information as possible. Please enjoy!

CHAPTER 1

WHAT IS APPLE CIDER VINEGAR?

New research has suggested that ingesting apple cider vinegar can fight diabetes, help people lose weight, lower blood pressure levels, and aid acid reflex problems.

The wonderful advantages of apple cider vinegar arise from its amazing compounds that heal, including the acetic acid mentioned in the introduction, along with enzymes, probiotics, magnesium, and potassium.

Raw, organic apple cider vinegar is an effective natural health supplement that can be used each day. You can use this to detox your body, help you digest the food you eat, and to get a fast energy burst that is healthier than coffee.

In addition, you can include apple cider vinegar into your personal care routine to whiten your teeth, make your hair softer, and even to clean your kitchen. Chapter three will cover other beauty benefits of this liquid in greater detail.

Regular vs. Raw Apple Cider Vinegar:

Apple cider vinegar (the unfiltered variety) can be made from water and apple juice, but in this case, it probably isn't pasteurized, and the "mother" has not yet been filtered out. It has a cloudy appearance and might have some sediment in the bottom of the bottle.

Killing the bad, Helping the Good Grow:

The acetic acid present in apple cider vinegar has the capability of killing off dangerous bacteria while also supporting the growth of healthy bacteria. Since this acid kills off dangerous bacteria as soon as it contacts it, it basically functions as a gentle, natural antibiotic for your body.

So apple cider vinegar can provide your body natural benefits in regards to higher immunity to diseases, digestion aid, and nicer skin without side effects. Of course, for some people, there may be exceptions. We will cover side effects and possible interactions later on in the book so you can stay safe.

A great Source of Polyphenols:

In addition to the benefits already mentioned, apple cider vinegar is a quality source for something called polyphenols. Studies support the fact that polyphenols can help to prevent cancer, diabetes, osteoporosis, cardiovascular issues, and diseases such as Alzheimer's.

Similar to Fermented Liquids:

Just like other fermented products, apple cider vinegar can be made using sugar combined with active yeast. When this happens, people use the naturally occurring source of sugar that crushed apples provide.

The sugar gets consumed by the yeast and uses it to create healthy bacteria, which is the process of fermentation in a nutshell.

Organic Sources:

The absolute best sources of apple cider vinegar for health, therapeutic, and wellness purposes should come from apples that are certified organic. Pasteurization isn't crucial and isn't even recommended if you want to use it for health-related reasons since pasteurization kills off the enzymes and delicate nutrients in the liquid.

The Prevention of Bad Bacteria:

Vinegar's acidity helps to prevent bad bacteria, such as E. Coli for example, from developing. Once the process of fermentation is complete, acetic acid has formed, the major advantageous compound present in apple cider vinegar.

<u>Unattractive Apple Cider Vinegar is a Good Sign:</u>

Some new users may be put off by the fact that apple cider vinegar can look murky and have strings that look like cobwebs inside them. However, this is a great sign!

The brown, murky appearance of apple cider vinegar, along with the yeast strands that you might see, can actually be an indication that the apple cider vinegar is high-quality liquid. The strands are live yeasts that are actually living. These strands have bacteria that will provide amazing health benefits once they enter your body.

Apple Cider Vinegar hardly has Sugar or Calories:

Though you make apple cider vinegar with sugar, the fermentation process causes the sugar to be consumed, so by the end product, you will hardly be ingesting any of it. Apple cider vinegar has between three and five calories for each tablespoon, and you only need a little to achieve the benefits you desire.

In other words, you end up with a great drink that has little to no sugar or calories. Actually, one major advantage to consuming apple cider vinegar is the positive impact on your blood sugar levels, as mentioned earlier. It helps them stay stable, reducing hypoglycemia and diabetes risks.

Apple Cider Vinegar as a Disinfectant:

Vinegar is proven to have abilities to fight fungus and to kill bad pathogens and bacteria. Throughout history, people have used it to clean their bodies, homes, and to prevent fungus. In modern day, people are still using apple cider vinegar extensively to clean their houses and bodies.

History and Overview of Apple Cider Vinegar

Did you know that apple cider vinegar has been ingested for over 2,000 years? Records of history prove that people have been fermenting apple juice into vinegar since around 5,000 BC or earlier.

Cleansing the Body:

Throughout time, apple cider vinegar has been put to use as a circulation stimulant a detoxification aid for the liver, a way to improve immunity, cleanse the lymph nodes, and to purify the blood. Actually, Hippocrates was known to prescribe apple cider vinegar for colds and coughs, mixed with a little honey.

How Else Did the Ancients Use Apple Cider Vinegar?

Vinegar, especially apple cider vinegar, is one of our greatest gifts from nature and the history of the liquid proves this. This vinegar is truly natural. All alcoholic beverages, whether made from plain sugar, rice, dates, grapes, or apples, will turn into vinegar after exposed to the air.

The bacteria present in the air is always there, and it converts alcohol from beer, wine, and cider into the previously mentioned acetic acid. This is what causes vinegar to taste so sour and sharp. Given this information, it's safe to assume that humans have been using vinegar since before they started recording that use.

The Recorded History of Vinegar:

The recorded history of vinegar begins at 5,000 BC. The Babylonians started using date palm fruit for creating vinegar and wine. This was used to pickle items, preserve food, and just to eat it. Residues from vinegar have been discovered in urns from ancient Egypt as old as 3,000 BC. In addition, the history of recorded vinegar use is present in texts from 1,200 BC in China.

Biblical Use of Vinegar:

In the times of the Bible, vinegar was being drunk for energy, used for medicine, and put on foods as flavoring. The liquid is mentioned in the new and old testaments of the bible. For instance, Ruth, after working hard in the barley fields, was given bread and vinegar by Boaz.

Vinegar and the Military:

The history of vinegar shows plenty of examples of the usefulness of the substance to soldiers. Vinegar, diluted in water, has been given as an energizing and strengthening tonic throughout history by the military.

"Posca" and Roman Soldiers:

Soldiers in ancient Roman times referred to this drink as "posca" and drank it often, just as the Japanese samurai did. Adding this substance to ordinary water also kills off infectious agents within the liquid, making it safer to drink.

Speeding up Healing:

Across history, vinegar has been recognized for its antiseptic nature and was used to disinfect and clean wounds of soldiers, speeding up their healing. Apple cider vinegar was also used in this way throughout the civil war in America, along with the times of World War One.

The Dissolving Abilities of Vinegar:

Vinegar has a well-known dissolving power that was used by Hannibal, the Carthaginian general when he went with elephants across the Alps and invaded Italy around the year 218 BC. This liquid was poured over hot stones to break them up, allowing his men to proceed and march across.

Vinegar and Louis XIII:

Louis XIII of France (who lived between 1601 and 1643) is said to have paid over a million Francs for vinegar so he could cool his army's cannons in a battle. Vinegar was applied to the cannons (made of hot iron) and cooled them down, preventing rust and cleaning the metal surface.

Vinegar in the Middle Ages:

Another use of apple cider vinegar in history was the Middle Ages. In addition to abrasive substances like sand, vinegar can be (and was) used to polish and clean armor.

Surprising Uses of Vinegar in History:

Cleopatra and Vinegar:

Around the year 40 BC, history says that the queen of Egypt, Cleopatra, won a bet with Mark Anthony, the Roman General, when she dissolved an expensive pearl in a glass of vinegar and drank it down. She had wagered that she could offer a feast for them both that cost a fortune.

Vinegar and Alchemy:

European alchemists were no stranger to vinegar around the Middle Ages. They poured vinegar over the lead, making a sweet substance known as sugar of lead. This substance was put to use for sweetening and smoothing out the taste of harsh cider.

Sadly, lead acetate is a poisonous subject and lead to the death of many cider drinkers in Europe around this time. Please note that you should never store vinegar in containers of crystal glass, iron, copper, or lead.

The Bubonic Plague:

From the 1300s to the 1700s, many cities in Europe were affected by the awful bubonic plague. At this time, around 50 million people perished due to this disease, which spread to men from rats and fleas.

By the year 1721, the plague had hit cities in France so hard that it was impossible to decently bury all of the dead. In order to solve this situation, authorities in the country let condemned convicts out of prison so they could help bury the bodies.

According to historical accords, most people died, but a particular group of convicted thieves survived by drinking garlic-infused vinegar every day in large amounts. Due to this, garlic-steeped vinegar is still known as Four Thieves Vinegar today.

European aristocrats held sponges soaked in vinegar to their noises to ward off the harmful odors of raw sewage and outdoor garbage in the 17th and 18th centuries. Vinaigrettes (small boxes) were carried around with these sponges inside, and many people stored these in their walking canes in special compartments.

Vinegar and Commercial Use:

In the late 1300s, some vintners in France came up with a method for creating vinegar known as the Orleans method. This involved using oak barrels to ferment the vinegar, then siphoning the liquid off using a spigot located on the barrel bottom.

About 15 percent of this liquid remained behind and had floating on top the famous "Mother of vinegar" along with concentrated bacteria. Then, a new batch of wine or cider was added to this barrel, which the remaining vinegar jump started for fermentation.

This group of vintners in France started a master vinegar creator's guild, using their Orleans method, and were able to supply the market of lucrative vinegar making.

Vinegar as Flavoring:

The industry of vinegar in the area was flourishing at the time of the Renaissance. Many kinds of vinegar flavored with flowers, fruits, herbs, and spices came out around this time, and around the 18th century, more than a hundred types existed.

Common Myths about Apple Cider Vinegar

Myth #1: Apple cider vinegar has identical nutrients as a normal apple.

Even though apple cider vinegar does come from apples being fermented, hard cider does too, and this doesn't lead people to drink it to gain more health. Apples have Vitamin C and fiber, but these are not present in apple cider vinegar. As mentioned, potassium does exist in the liquid, but only about 5 percent of how much there is of a real apple.

Myth #2: Apple cider vinegar offers no health advantages.

A lot of people believe that apple cider vinegar cannot possibly have so many health benefits. As you will see throughout this book, it clearly does!

Myth #3: All Apple cider vinegar is created equal.

When it comes to cheap brands to more expensive, better organic types, it appears as though nearly all food companies are trying to get the apple cider vinegar kick and profit from it.

However, there are differences between types of apple cider vinegar. The clear types have been thoroughly processed and filtered, sacrificing some of its amazing health benefits. Instead, go for the murky-looking, brown variety if possible.

Myth #4: You can only use it to drink or eat.

With the health advantages touted for apple cider vinegar, it appears as though this is as far as its benefits go. However, it's a very versatile liquid. Apple cider vinegar is great for cleaning the house because of its antimicrobial functions. Use it to wipe your counters at home, and you'll be amazed.

Myth #5: You should never use apple cider vinegar topically.

Due to its strong smell and acidic components, apple cider vinegar seems as though it would be too harsh to use on your skin, but this is not the case. It shouldn't be used to replace your facial moisturizer, but when you mix it with water, you can use it for a facial toner to clear makeup and dirt away from your face.

To do this, simply apply the apple cider vinegar to your face using a cotton swab and keep it there for 10 minutes, then rinse it off. This mixture can be used to replace your ordinary face wash, but only do it about three times each week.

Myth #6: Apple cider vinegar is the only type of vinegar that is healthy.

Apple cider vinegar is very healthy and is considered the best of the best, but some health advantages can be reaped from other types of vinegar, as well. Since all vinegar has acetic acid in it, plain white vinegar and balsamic vinegar can also be beneficial.

Myth #7: Apple cider vinegar is only fit for human use.

Your pet can actually benefit from this liquid, as well. In fact, some holistic veterinarians use it to fix itchy ears and skin in animals. Just use equal parts water and apple cider vinegar, then spray it onto your dog or cat's itchy spots to bring relief. Never spray this onto open wounds.

Myth #8: It doesn't taste good.

Some people like the taste of apple cider vinegar and others don't. It's true that taste is an individual preference and is very subjective, but you don't have to take apple cider vinegar by itself. You can mix it with melted coconut or olive oil and herbs to create a tasty salad dressing or mix it into a fruit smoothie.

Later on in the book, we will cover some specific recipes you can use to get the benefits of apple cider vinegar without drinking it by itself.

CHAPTER 2

HOW TO MAKE RAW APPLE CIDER VINEGAR

When apple season comes around, it's time to create your own apple cider vinegar at home. If you can't find a locally grown source for apples where you live, you can just buy a bag from your local store (make sure they're organic though).

Why Make Your Own?

Raw, unpasteurized apple cider vinegar costs a lot, so you can save money by making your own at home. Your average quart of the liquid will cost you around $5 at the majority of health grocery stores.

You can create an entire gallon or more for this price, or even cheaper using apple scraps that would've been thrown away anyway.

Which Apples to Use:

You might be wondering which types of apples to use to make your homemade apple cider vinegar. The truth is that a mix of apples is what will create the healthiest and best-tasting type. If you have never done this before, try out the ratios below to create your very first batch, and you can mix it as you prefer later on.

- 50 Percent sweet types of apples, such as Red Delicious, Fuji, or Golden Delicious.

- About 35 percent sharp apples, like Liberty, Northern Spy, or Liberty.

- 15 percent bitter apples, like Cortland, Porter's Perfection, or Newtown.

In some places, bitter apples might be hard to find at the store. If you encounter this problem, you can use 60 percent sweet apples and use 40 percent sharp apples. The flavor won't end up being as complex, but it will work just fine. If you just have one type of apple tree at home, though, you can just use that type to create your apple cider vinegar.

Making Raw ACV at Home:

This recipe will make about a gallon of apple cider vinegar but can be adjusted to suit your needs. For example, use half to get half the amount, and twice the amount to get twice as much.

Plus, you can make as much as you want without having to go buy more. Who can argue with that type of convenience? When you make your own, you get to control the quality, the process of making it, and how much to create. Keep reading to find out how to make this amazing liquid to help your health.

Your Ingredients List:

- Five big apples, or the leftovers from 10 apples.
- Clean, filtered water.
- Organic sugar or raw honey (1 cup).
- 1 Gallon jar made of glass.
- One large rubber band.
- A cheesecloth for straining.

Instructions for making Raw ACV:

Before you start this process, you need to create hard apple cider, first. The alcohol from this mixture is what causes acetic acid to form, which is what contributes to the sour taste and health benefits of apple cider vinegar. Then, you're ready to follow these steps:

1. Make sure your apples are washed, then chop it up into coarse pieces of about an inch across. The seeds, stems, and cores can be included in this.

2. Put your coarsely chopped apple pieces in your jar (after making sure it's clean). Make sure you aren't brewing this cider in steel pots since the acidic mixture can cause heavy metals to leach and harm your body. The apples should fill the jar at least halfway or more. Add more scraps and chunks until the jar is at least halfway full.

3. Pour water over the scraps and apple chunks until they are covered, and your container is almost full, but leave some room toward the top. Make sure the water is room temperature.

4. Stir the sugar and honey into the container until it dissolves completely. Cover your jar with a cheesecloth and hold it in place with a big rubber band.

5. Leave this jar sitting on your counter for a week or two, but remember to mix it gently a couple of times each day. You will notice bubbles forming. This is the sugar being fermented into an alcohol substance. You will also notice this in the smell of the mixture.

6. You will know that the hard cider is ready when the chunks of apple don't float anymore and have sunk to the jar's bottom. If the apple chunks still have not sunk down after 14 days but your mix smells like alcohol, move onto the following step.

7. Strain the apple chunks out, pouring the resulting liquid to a clean jar or multiple smaller jars. Then, cover this with a new cheesecloth, tying it on using a rubber band.

8. Leave this mixture on your counter for another three to four weeks so that the alcohol can get transformed into acetic acid by the acetic acid bacteria. Seeing some sediment at the jar's bottom is to be expected. You will

see the mother culture start to form on the top of the liquid.

9. You can taste your mixture after three weeks to see if it's done If the taste seems right for you, strain the mix and keep it in clean jugs or mason jars. If the taste doesn't seem right after four weeks, leave it for seven days and make another attempt.

10. If you forget about it and it's left too long, you may strain the mix and dilute it with water until it reaches the level you want.

This mixture can be used as you pleased but be sure to store it way from sunlight or extreme temperatures.

Raw, organic apple cider vinegar will not go bad, but another mother will form atop it if it's left for too long, so keep that in mind. If this does happen, it's fine, you will just need to restrain it and dilute again if it's too strong tasting.

Remember that your homemade vinegar isn't just useful for the kitchen. You can also use it in the bath (add two cups to a tub full of water) to help your body detox. You may also use it as a compress when you get a bruise or sprain, as people once did before ice was more common.

Remember to use Non-Pasteurized:

As mentioned before, apple cider vinegar that has been pasteurized doesn't give you the same health advantages as the raw stuff in terms of enzymes, probiotics, or vitamins. If you decide to go through the process of making your own apple cider vinegar, make sure it's raw.

Don't use Plastic Packaged Apple Cider Vinegar:

Another issue with apple cider vinegar that has been pasteurized is that it's often packaged in a plastic bottle. The acidic apple cider vinegar will leach chemicals from the plastic into the fluid. If you make your own or buy it at the store, always make sure it's a glass bottle.

More Uses for Apple Cider Vinegar to Know about:

The uses for this liquid are seemingly endless. You can make a master tonic with it, which is a natural anti-viral and anti-flu agent. Apple cider vinegar is also an important component of bone broth. Let's look at some other uses for this liquid.

Polishing Wood:

Apple cider vinegar can actually be used to condition wood. Just mix half a cup of the fluid with half a cup of oil (such as olive or vegetable), and it will create a great furniture polish for removing water stains and treating surfaces.

Treating Digestion Issues:

If you drink a bit before eating, apple cider vinegar will treat digestion issues such as indigestion and bloating.

Curing Warts:

Although the scientific proof for this is not very vast, there are countless testimonials online that swear by using apple cider vinegar to cure warts. Before going to bed, soak a cotton swab with some diluted apple cider vinegar and paste it in place overnight. Your wart may throb and swell, then fall off after a couple weeks.

An Alternative to Harsh Chemicals:

A lot of people don't like the idea of spraying their home with harsh chemicals. Get rid of the commercial stuff and make your own with two parts water to one-part vinegar. You may add some essential oils for scent and extra disinfectant properties.

<u>A Word from the Experts:</u>

Dr. Sandi Rogers, a naturopath CEO of a College of Traditional Medicine in Australia, has been studying the healing benefits of apple cider vinegar for over three decades and believes that it's an impressive medicine. Rogers believes that the superfood status of apple cider vinegar is due to its high content of minerals.

Since minerals are so foundational to wellbeing and health (not vitamins, as some believe), taking this liquid each day can help you immensely, especially with mineral absorption from your diet.

How much to Use:

Use regular, small amounts, such as a couple teaspoons dissolved in some water. Swish it around in your mouth in order to activate your salivary glands.

The Safety of Apple Cider Vinegar:

Many may wonder, is apple cider vinegar completely safe? Admittedly, the risks and benefits of this liquid aren't completely known yet, so if you have any doubts, your illnesses should always be managed and treated with a professional of medical status.

Again, the uglier the vinegar, the healthier it is. For most people, drinking apple cider vinegar straight will be too sour to handle and may even burn the esophagus. For this reason, dilute it with water. If you still can't stand the sourness, add some raw honey to the water before drinking.

All about "The Mother"

You have heard us mention "the mother" a couple of times, but what exactly does this mean? Again, it's crucial to realize that apple cider vinegar can vary greatly in quality. In order to get the best of the best apple cider vinegar, make sure the mother is still intact in the bottle.

The mother ensures that the vinegar still has its advantageous components, such as probiotics. The mother probiotics are the cloudy strands within the vinegar where all of the health benefits come from.

AMAZING Health Benefits of Apple Cider Vinegar

After reading this far, you should have a pretty good understanding of why you should use apple cider vinegar on a daily basis. But here are some more health benefits to be aware of:

- **Body Detox:** Raw, unfiltered apple cider vinegar is a lymphatic and liver tonic which helps your body clean itself out, balancing the pH, stimulating bowel motility, cardiovascular stimulation, and lymphatic drainage. In other words, it really helps your body get clean!

- Usually, when we hear the word acid, associated with vinegar, we automatically assume that acid is bad. However, for this, acid is very good. Similar to the way lemon juice contains citric acid which helps lemon water detoxify your body, the acetic acid in apple cider vinegar also has an incredible alkalizing effect on you. This aids in weight loss efforts, energy levels, and many other things.

- **Teeth Whitening:** Apple cider vinegar has a high pH level which is useful for removing stains, not just from your kitchen counters, but from your teeth. Just take your first finger, dip it in some apple cider vinegar and rub it onto your

- teeth, allowing it to sit for one to two minutes.

- **Treating Heartburn and Acid Reflux:** One of the main reasons that people get acid reflux and uncomfortable heartburn is a stomach pH that isn't balanced enough, lacking probiotics and important enzymes. Luckily, apple cider vinegar has plenty of these essential nutrients.

- How should this be taken? Just add a tablespoon of the liquid to a full glass of water and make sure to drink it down five to 10 minutes before eating. This will relieve your heartburn and acid reflux symptoms.

- **Killing Candida:** Countless people across the globe struggle with yeast and candida. This can lead to digestive problems, UTIs, a lack of energy, and bad breath. Thankfully, apple cider vinegar has properties to help this.

- The probiotics present in apple cider vinegar will help promote probiotic growth to kill this harmful yeast. Another way to help this is to stop eating sugar altogether.

- **Keep your pH Levels Balanced:** Apple cider vinegar, as stated a few times already, is full of acetic acid, which has an alkalizing effect on your body. Keeping your pH in balance will help reduce the risk of cancer and improve your energy levels.

- **Supports Metabolism:** A research study done by the *Journal of Diabetes Care* discovered that you could promote weight loss by ingesting apple cider vinegar. A few different reasons exist for this, but one main reason is that apple cider vinegar reduces cravings for sugar and helps detox your body.

- Another useful study discovered that adding acetic acid to the diet reduced the body fat of rats by up to 10 percent. Another study done in 2005 discovered that consuming vinegar along with a meal with high carbs reduced the drinking and eating of participants by 200 to 275 calories within a day.

- **Ease your Sunburn:** Sunburn can be very uncomfortable, but apple cider vinegar is here to the rescue again! Just add a cup of the liquid to a mildly temperature bath with some lavender essential oil and a quarter cup of coconut oil. This will help your sunburn not only feel better in the moment, but heal overall.

- **Balance your Blood Sugar:** Studies have shown that acetic acid helps to balance blood sugar, improving insulin responses and sensitivity.

- **Soothing Inflammation and Swelling:** Raw, organic apple cider vinegar has potassium in it, which helps to reduce inflammation and swelling. This can be used to treat poison ivy.

- **Get Fleas off your Dog or Cat:** An apple cider vinegar solution can help remove fleas from your pets. Just mix together 50 percent water with 50 percent apple cider vinegar and wash your pet with the mix. Do this once per day for a few weeks, and your pet will be free from fleas.

- **Help Allergies:** Yet another great way to use apple cider vinegar is to treat allergies. Apple cider vinegar can help to break the mucous up in your body. In addition, it clears sinuses and supports a healthy immune system. You can drink it a few times a day to cure your allergy symptoms.

- **Kill Toenail Fungus:** The antifungal and antibacterial components of apple cider vinegar will help kill toenail and skin fungus. Just rub some apple cider vinegar onto the affected area a couple times a day.

- **Fight Eczema:** As mentioned, apple cider vinegar has a high pH level, making it great for curing skin problems. Next time your eczema pops up, rub the liquid onto the affected area or wash with it. You can also use essential oils and coconut oil to heal further.

- **Fight Varicose Veins:** This miracle liquid is great for fighting varicose veins. This is possible because apple cider vinegar improves your circulation, is anti-inflammatory, and supports the health of your vein walls, reducing the bulging veins. Just mix the liquid with some witch hazel, then rub it onto your veins to see improvement.

- **A Sore Throat Cure:** Due to its probiotic properties and vitamins, apple cider vinegar is a great way to cure your sore throat or cold. Take a spoonful diluted in water thrice daily to have this effect.

- **Fight Odors:** Harmful yeast and bad bacteria are a couple of the main causes of bad body odors. Your armpits often stay damp throughout the day, leading to bad bacteria and the smell we associate with that area.

- Just dabbing some of your homemade, raw apple cider vinegar under this area can help to neutralize odors by killing off the yeast there.

Scientific Backed Claims of Apple Cider Vinegar

Even after reading this far into the book, you might still be skeptical about whether apple cider vinegar really can offer all these amazing benefits. So for this section, we are going to focus primarily on scientifically-backed claims of the health benefits of apple cider vinegar.

Fosters Healthy Cholesterol in the Body:

Apple cider vinegar can not only support your body's cholesterol levels, but research has proven that it also protects your body from oxidation or arterial damage, which high cholesterol can lead to. WebMD mentions a study done in the mid 2000's that provided evidence for apple cider vinegar lowering cholesterol numbers

Reduces Water Retention:

We've already mentioned that apple cider vinegar is a helpful weight loss aid, but did you know that it also reduces water retention? Paired with its abilities to increase your metabolism and suppress your appetite, this is a pretty amazing combination for those looking to shed some extra weight. The Journal of Agricultural and Food Chemistry found out in 2010 that apple cider vinegar reduced water retention in mice.

Blocks Starch Digestion in the Body:

Research has proven that apple cider vinegar contains powerful anti-glycemic compounds that help your body support healthy levels of blood sugar. In addition, apple cider vinegar blocks starch digestion in your body (partially), which is known to raise blood sugar levels. A 2004 study done by "Diabetes Care" found a link between improved sensitivity to insulin and the consumption of vinegar, especially during high-carb meals.

Antioxidants:

Apple cider vinegar has multiple antioxidants which will help you stay physically healthy and keep your body running in top shape. Biochem Pharmacol published a paper in 1994 that discovered high antioxidant activity in the acetic acid present in apple cider vinegar.

Helps you Absorb Vegetable Nutrients:

We've already mentioned that the acetic acid present in this vinegar helps your body absorb crucial nutrients from your food, but did you know that adding some of this to your salad can specifically help you get the most out of your vegetables and leafy greens?

Researchers in Japan, working for Biosci Biotechnol chemistry found that dietary vinegar helped the intestinal absorption of calcium in rats in 1999

Fights Diabetes:

The next incredible advantage that apple cider vinegar offers is that it can become part of a great plan to help diabetes. Multiple studies have discovered that apple cider vinegar can lower your levels of glucose, meaning that it's an effective treatment for those suffering from type 2 diabetes.

A study done in 2007 by the University of Arizona discovered that drinking two tablespoons of the liquid in addition to 30 grams of cheese right before going to sleep could decrease fasting levels of blood sugar by 4 to 6 percent!

Another study done by *Diabetes Care,* the medical journal, discovered that taking just two tablespoons of the liquid before a meal can decrease levels of blood sugar by 6 percent! That's because the liquid has been proven to reduce A1C levels and balance out levels of blood sugar, which helps diabetics immensely.

In addition, if you eat and typically experience a spike in blood sugar afterward, the vinegar can help your energy levels rise again.

CHAPTER 3

DETOXING WITH APPLE CIDER VINEGAR

We have already covered some of the incredible benefits of apple cider vinegar, including its ability to lower your blood pressure, treat acid reflux, and support the overall health of your gut. In addition, the acetic acid within apple cider vinegar helps to support healthy digestive function, and only a little is needed to reap these benefits.

Let's look next at one of the greatest benefits of apple cider vinegar, its role in effective weight loss.

Natural Weight Loss using Apple Cider Vinegar:

Being overweight is embarrassing in addition to being uncomfortable. If you have been trying and trying to lose weight and keep it off, you're probably ready to try something completely new.

Apple Cider Vinegar and Dieting:

ACV (apple cider vinegar) is a well-known natural remedy and is used by countless people to both cure and prevent common ailments. In addition, this liquid holds a crucial spot in the world of dieting. Scientific research along with personal experiences have proven that apple cider vinegar can, in fact, help you reach your ideal weight.

The Long-Term Answer:

Just treating the symptoms of a problem, without going deeper, will not provide a lasting solution. Apple cider vinegar is a substance that can target your weight problem from a holistic perspective, offering a long-term answer instead of a quick fix.

Proof and Research about ACV and Weight Loss:

This chapter is here to help you know how apple cider vinegar works, along with how you can use it day to day to improve your overall health and lose that extra weight.

One of the most interesting studies done on how this liquid can aid weight loss was done in the year 2009 by *Bioscience, Biotechnology, and Biochemistry.* This study found that drinking a couple of tablespoons of apple cider vinegar for a few months caused participants to lose significant amounts of body fat and waist circumference.

How does Apple Cider Vinegar help your Body Shed Weight?

Apple cider vinegar comes from apples that are crushed, distilled, and finally fermented, as we went over earlier in the book. This results in acetic acid, a liquid that taps into some important physiological functions and supports the healthy loss of extra weight on your body. Let's look at some of the other reasons it helps you lose weight.

The Appetite Suppressant Effect:

Apple cider vinegar, first and foremost, helps you to eat less, causing your body to feel satisfied sooner than it normally would while eating. One study that showed this beyond doubt was done in 2005. The participants who ate their bread with some vinegar got full faster than the others who ate just bread.

The higher amount of acetic acid they consumed, the fuller the participants felt over the course of the study.

Blood Sugar Control for Weight Loss:

Apple cider vinegar helps to control your levels of blood sugar, as mentioned previously. It prevents those uncontrollable spikes in sugar and the crashes that lead you to want to snack in between the main meals of the day.

Once your blood sugar levels are stable, you will find it easier to eat just when you're hungry and stay with your diet. The study mentioned before also kept track of blood sugar levels with both the control group and vinegar group.

Study participants who consumed apple cider vinegar had much lower blood glucose levels after their meal. In other words, there wasn't the spike that usually comes after a high-carb meal. In addition, the ones who consumed larger doses of apple cider vinegar were still benefiting from the impact an hour and a half after they ate.

It helps to Prevent the Accumulation of Fat:

Apple cider vinegar helps to stimulate your body's metabolism function which helps you burn more fat faster. In addition, it has a lot of enzyme and organic acids that help you burn more fat by speeding your metabolism up.

Insulin Secretion and Apple Cider Vinegar:

Did you know that insulin plays a role in your body's storage of fat? It's true. Insulin is closely related to your levels of blood sugar, and the secretion of this hormone is disrupted in those who suffer from diabetes (type 2).

Some scientists suggested that apple cider vinegar could work very similarly to diabetic drugs, controlling this disease. For helping to cure your diabetes, diet is highly important. Do plenty of research into the foods and spices you should be consuming.

Apple Cider Vinegar's Detoxing Effect and Weight Loss:

When your body sheds harmful toxins, metabolism and digestion become much more efficient than before. Apple cider vinegar flushes out your body, allowing it to make the best use of the nutrients you eat. It also has high levels of insoluble fiber, improving bowel movements and absorbing toxins.

Which Type of Apple Cider Vinegar to Use for Losing Weight:

We've gone over this for other health benefits of apple cider vinegar, but it's especially crucial for weight loss. When you are using the liquid for this specific purpose, it must be raw and unprocessed. Better yet, use the kind you are making at home.

You should know by now that you should only be using apple cider vinegar that still has the mother intact to get the best benefits possible.

Avoiding Pesticides:

Apples are one of the most heavily sprayed fruits out there, when it comes to pesticides, making organic choices very important! You must purchase unfiltered, unprocessed, raw apple cider vinegar to get the benefits you seek and to lose weight, or just make your own.

Brand isn't as Important as Other Factors:

You may be wondering which brand of apple cider vinegar to use for weight loss, but brand doesn't matter as much as some other considerations. Any apple cider vinegar brand that is organic, unfiltered, and unpasteurized may be used for this reason.

One very common brand of organic apple cider vinegar is Bragg. You can buy this on the Internet, in health food stores, or in ordinary supermarkets, sometimes.

Don't worry about the apple cider vinegar not being pasteurized, since vinegar has a high enough level of acidity to kill off E. Coli and other harmful bacteria. Keep in mind that many doctors say that pregnant women shouldn't consume unpasteurized foods.

Steps for Using ACV to Lose Weight:

For those who don't like or are not accustomed to the flavor and impact of apple cider vinegar, you can start by including the liquid gradually in your diet, being careful not to use too much. This will prevent adverse effects.

How to Start:

You can begin by adding just a teaspoon of the vinegar to a glass of water, drinking this mixture at least one time per day. You can slowly increase the amount every time and how often you drink it.

The Optimal Amount to Drink:

According to studies on apple cider vinegar and weight loss, the ideal amount to consume per day is two tablespoons, diluted in water. Dilution is important because the liquid is highly acidic and dilution helps to protect your stomach lining, throat, and teeth.

Using a Straw:

Don't ever drink apple cider vinegar undiluted, this will cause you more harm than anything else. You may drink the diluted mix of apple cider vinegar and water using a straw. This will keep your tooth enamel safe.

Using Honey with Apple Cider Vinegar:

Some people will discover that the apple cider vinegar taste is hard to stand. In order to make the flavor more tolerable, you may add a little honey to it. The honey will mix better if you use warm water.

Mixing apple cider vinegar and honey have benefits for your health, and it also tastes great. If you are aiming to lose weight, try not to use too much honey as sugar can get in the way of weight loss.

Adding Apple Cider Vinegar to Food:

- **Soups**: Apple cider vinegar can be used with certain foods and goes especially well with meat or bean soups. Just keep in mind that you should add the vinegar to your food after it has cooled. This will prevent the loss of nutrients to the heat.

- **Salads**: Apple cider vinegar is a popular dressing for salads and tastes especially great with olive oil and herbs added.

- **Pickling**: For those who enjoy pickles or similar flavors, you can use apple cider vinegar to pickle cucumbers or other vegetables.

- **Herbal Tea**: For those who don't mind the taste of apple cider vinegar, you can add it to your herbal teas to get the health benefits. This book will go over some other recipes later on.

How Often Should You Drink it?

In order to jump-start your metabolism and get the benefits of feeling full, some say that you must drink diluted apple cider vinegar an hour before eating to help you lose weight and improve digestion.

Morning Vinegar:

Some swear by drinking their apple cider vinegar right when they wake up and have empty stomachs. But others prefer not to do this. If you aren't comfortable drinking it without food in your stomach, you can do it after meals.

After Meals:

If you're more comfortable consuming apple cider vinegar after meals, you can do this two to three times per day. If you feel nausea or burning in your stomach, reduce how much you're taking.

Taking Breaks:

Some people recommend not consuming apple cider vinegar every single day and making sure to take breaks every month or so. As you can see, it all depends on what suits you best.

Possible Side Effects of Apple Cider Vinegar:

ACV is considered generally safe for human consumption, but as with all traditional remedies, you should take some precautions to make sure you're safe. Too much apple cider vinegar could lead to lowered levels of potassium in the body, causing osteoporosis.

But this effect happened to someone who drank 8 oz. of ACV every day for multiple years in a row. As you can see, we recommend jutting a couple tablespoons diluted every day, which is more than safe to consume regularly.

As said before, acidic items like apple cider vinegar can lead to weaker tooth enamel, so to prevent that, just rinse the mouth out with water each time you drink the apple cider vinegar mixture. Use a straw, too, to prevent tooth problems. You might also wish to refrain from brushing your teeth right after taking your apple cider vinegar mix.

Asking your Doctor about Interactions:

Apple cider vinegar may interact with diabetes medications, heart medications, laxatives, or diuretics. If you're on any meds, make sure you ask your physician before you decide to drink apple cider vinegar regularly.

Why is Apple Cider Vinegar Superior to Other Types for Losing Weight?

Apple cider vinegar is believed to be the best choice when it comes to weight loss, due to all of the health advantages it offers. It will clean your body, offering anti-microbial effects.

Considering the fact that it can aid high blood pressure, heart issues, diabetes, digestion, acid reflux, and possibly even kidney stones, it's obvious why apple cider vinegar is the best type of vinegar to use for health reasons.

What Should You Expect Using Apple Cider Vinegar To Lose Weight?

Apple cider vinegar should not be expected to give you an instant cure for a weight problem. The changes you see will happen on a gradual basis, but they will be permanent.

Patience is Key:

Remember to be patient, letting it work. At times, losing a pound per month and keeping it off is the real path to success. Don't get impatient and give up!

Other Factors in Weight Loss:

Also, keep in mind that the rate at which you lose your weight does depend on your other lifestyle habits, like genetics, stress, nutrition, and how much you exercise.

Making the Apple Cider Vinegar Work Better and Faster:

To get the fastest and best results, you have to combine this remedy with other proven methods. That way, the apple cider vinegar will work along with these other changes and give you the results you're hoping for.

Avoid Processed Foods:

If you're hoping to lose weight, you must avoid processed foods, unhealthy fats, and sugar. All of these will counteract the effects of the vinegar.

Find some Exercise You Enjoy:

Even moving moderately up to five times each week can help you speed up your metabolism and lose weight faster. Start by walking for 10 minutes each day and work your way up.

Potassium-Rich Foods:

If you eat foods that have plenty of potassium, this mineral can lower your blood pressure and reduce your stress levels. Each more spinach, avocados, sweet potatoes, and bananas to get this effect.

<u>Beauty Benefits of Apple Cider Vinegar:</u>

Apple cider vinegar isn't just good for your health and cleaning, it also has beauty benefits that help you look better! Let's look at some of those now.

Beauty Benefit #1: Use it to Brighten Your Nails.

Stained or yellow nails can be a bit embarrassing, and this occurs from smoking or other tasks. It can happen after working with dyes or chemicals or just bad habits. Whatever your reason for having stained nails, apple cider vinegar can help whiten them.

The acetic and malic acids present in apple cider vinegar will reduce the stains on your nails and also help to treat nail infections, which can lead to discoloration. Here are the steps for cleaning your nails with apple cider vinegar:

- Put half a cup of lukewarm water and half a cup of apple cider vinegar into a bowl wide enough to soak your hands in.

- Soak your yellowed nails in the mixture for up to a half hour, then rise.

- Use coconut or olive oil to massage into each nail.

- You can do this twice a day until your nails brighten up.

Beauty Benefit #2: Keep Pimples and Acne Away.

If you have a pimple problem, apple cider vinegar can help with that, as well. The liquid has antibacterial and antiseptic properties that help keep pimples away by freeing your pores of dust particles, oil, and bacteria.

It also helps your skin regain a healthy pH balance, which helps to keep breakouts away. Here are the steps for using apple cider vinegar to treat and prevent acne:

- Mix two parts water with one-part organic apple cider vinegar in a bowl.

- Wet some cotton balls with the liquid, putting it on your affected area.

- Let this sit for 15 minutes and then rinse it.

- You can do this up to three times per day for four days.

Beauty Benefit #3: Use it for Skin Toning.

People with oily skin can benefit from apple cider vinegar due to its properties that work as an astringent. Apple cider vinegar contains properties that help get more blood flow going on your face, minimizing pores.

After a short time, your skin will start looking much better. Just stick with it faithfully so you can start to see the results you hope for. This, in combination with its antiseptic properties, it will help your skin look awesome. Just follow these steps to get the benefits:

- Mix half a cup of distilled water with half a cup of apple cider vinegar. You can add some essential oil too, like ylang-ylang or lavender, just use a few drops.

- Put this mixture on your face with a cotton ball, allowing it to sit three minutes.

- Rinse your face off using cold water. This can be done two times each day but make sure you shake the liquid before applying it.

For those with average skin, you can use two parts water with one-part apple cider vinegar for your toner, but if your skin is very sensitive, more water is suggested. Always make sure you test this out on a small area of your skin before using.

Keep in mind that when you use this liquid, the vinegar smell may stay on your skin for a bit, but does fade once the toner dries.

Beauty Benefit #4: Get Rid of Razor Burn and Bumps.

The irritated, small bumps you get on your skin after shaving are not only unattractive, but they can be painful. In order to help solve this issue, you may utilize apple cider vinegar.

The anti-inflammatory compounds in the apple cider vinegar will help soothe your irritated areas, reducing itching and inflammation. In addition to this, the acetic acid present in apple cider vinegar will soften your skin while keeping infections away, helping your ingrown hairs disappear.

In order to utilize this wonderful natural remedy for razor bumps and burn, follow these steps:

- Smear a small amount of honey over your razor burn, letting it sit for five minutes or so.

- Rinse the honey off using cool water.

- Using a cotton swab, put apple cider vinegar on the affected area, allowing it to try out on its own.

- This treatment can be repeated three times daily until your razor burn goes away.

Keep in mind that if you have sensitive skin, diluting the apple cider vinegar will be safer for you.

Beauty Benefit #5: Get rid of Teeth Stains.

If your teeth are yellow and stained, it can be embarrassing, making you self-conscious, but you can use apple cider vinegar to help clean them up. Discoloration comes from drinking too much coffee or smoking.

Apple cider vinegar's acetic acid content will help get rid of this yellow, stained surface, destroying harmful mouth bacteria and contributing to a healthier mouth all around. Here's how to use it for this:

- Mix a tablespoon of water with a tablespoon of apple cider vinegar and use it as a mouthwash in the morning and at night.

Beauty Benefit #6: Get rid of Dandruff.

Although dandruff isn't dangerous, it doesn't look very nice and can lead to embarrassment. This problem is worst during the winter because the air tends to be so dry.

Dandruff leads to dead, oily skin pieces on your hair and scalp. This may eventually cause a scaly, itchy head and even shoulders covered in dandruff flakes. ACV has antifungal compounds that restore your scalp's pH balance, cleaning out your hair follicles and clogged pores.

Here's how to use apple cider vinegar as a remedy for dandruff:

- Mix two tablespoons of water with two tablespoons of apple cider vinegar.

- Mix 15 drops of the liquid of tea tree oil.

- Spread this liquid onto your head, massaging for about five minutes, then let it sit for five minutes.

- Your hair can be rinsed and washed with shampoo as normal, and this treatment may be used three times each week until your issue is resolved.

Beauty Benefit #7: Make your Feet Smell Better.

Smelly feet, or foot odor, is an issue that is quite common but can still be unpleasant and embarrassing both for you and your friends. The antimicrobial properties of apple cider vinegar can help to disinfect and clean your feet, killing off bacteria that causes this odor.

Here are the steps you must take to kill foot odor using apple cider vinegar:

- Add five cups of warm water with a cup of apple cider vinegar.

- Let your feet sit in this liquid for up to 15 minutes.

- After you let them sit, wash them with water and soap.

- This can be used at home every day for about a month.

Beauty Benefit #8: Help your Sunburn Heal.

The sun is good for us in moderation, but when you're outside underneath it for too long, it can cause a painful sunburn. This turns your skin painful and red from the damage. In extreme cases, you might even get blisters.

Apple cider vinegar has been used for many years to cure this issue. Due to its natural astringent abilities, apple cider vinegar helps to speed healing and soothe the burning feeling. It also reduces inflammation and irritation.

Here's how to use apple cider vinegar to soothe your sunburn:

- Mix some cool water with an equal amount of apple cider vinegar, massaging this mixture onto your burn. This can be done a few times each day until the burn gets better.

- You may also take a lukewarm bath with a couple cups of apple cider vinegar into the tub to heal your burn. You can take two baths per day until your burn gets better.

As you can see, there are many different ways to use apple cider vinegar for beauty reasons.

CHAPTER 4

NATURAL CURES WITH APPLE CIDER VINEGAR

Apple cider vinegar, as you should know by now, is a highly versatile liquid and can be used for your health, cleaning, and as food. Natural health enthusiasts everywhere celebrate the healing abilities of apple cider vinegar for nearly every problem.

This chapter will cover how you can use apple cider vinegar to detox and cleanse your body.

The Miraculous Cleansing Abilities of ACV:

Using apple cider vinegar can help you clean your body because of its content of enzymes, vitamins, and minerals. It will detox your body, removing toxic waste and getting rid of bacteria before it can cause a lot of bodily damage to you.

Apple cider vinegar both improves bowel movement and aids digestion, detoxifying your liver, improving your body's circulation, and purifying your blood. It has strong enzymes that help to break down harmful cholesterol and keep it from clogging up your body and arteries.

How else does it Help your Body Detox?

Apple cider vinegar helps to maintain a positive alkaline pH balance to keep away inflammation in your body. Inflammation is caused by high levels of acid.

Apple cider vinegar also helps to clean your lymph nodes and break up the mucus present in your body, which then improves your immune system and lymph circulation. We've already covered the ways that apple cider vinegar can aid you with weight loss.

It allows your body to more effectively break fast down, rather than storing them on your body. It's also full of pectin to keep you fuller for longer, reducing water retention and suppressing an overactive appetite. If you combine apple cider vinegar with the right nutrition and exercise, it can help tremendously with keeping the fat away.

As mentioned before, selecting the right kind of this vinegar is a must for achieving the results you dream of. True apple cider vinegar is created by a fermentation process that turns apples into vinegar.

<u>Simple Apple Cider Recipes Anyone can do:</u>

Never choose pasteurized vinegar or the type that comes in a plastic bottle. Each time you use your organic apple cider vinegar, don't forget that you should shake the glass every time in order to get as many good elements as you can.

Using apple cider vinegar Internally:

Apple cider vinegar is highly acidic, so make sure you dilute it with water before drinking so your esophagus and teeth stay safe. Even though apple cider vinegar is acidic, it does create an alkaline effect in your body when ingested.

The fact that this liquid has an alkalizing impact on your body has a large effect on its abilities to heal so many ailments.

Don't Use too much:

You should never use too much of this liquid, just dilute a couple of tablespoons in a big glass with water, drinking it before or during meals twice per day.

Ingesting apple cider vinegar in typical food amounts is mostly very safe, as long as you don't use too much. Drinking too much of this daily could lead to health issues like a lower bone density or lowered levels of potassium.

In addition, apple cider vinegar can cause interactions with some medications, so ask your doctor before taking it with heart meds or diuretics.

An Eternal Apple Cider Vinegar Bath:

The skin is your biggest organ and has a lot to do with how effectively your body can detox. Although not everybody enjoys steam rooms or can access them, you may begin to cleanse your body at home in the tub.

True, not everyone likes the smell of apple cider vinegar, but its benefits are so plentiful that it's worth it. If you're very bothered by the scent, just add some essential oils to your bath. You may also add some herbs.

- Just add the raw apple cider vinegar to your tub, then let it soak in there for a minimum of 15 minutes. This is highly effective for fighting skin irritation and bacterial infections because of its antimicrobial benefits.

- This bath can be taken two times per week to help balance your skin's pH level and cause softer, nicer skin.

Making your Own Apple Cider Vinegar Detox Beverages:

Not everyone can stand the taste of apple cider vinegar diluted with just water, so if you're one of these people, you will surely appreciate the following recipes.

An Apple Cider Vinegar and Lemon Drink:

Lemon water is another liquid that helps immensely with weight management, digestion, and other health issues. This beverage has some cinnamon in it, too, which metabolizes glucose in your body to help prevent the storage of fat.

Cinnamon also aids your digestion to help you feel full and stay that way for much longer. The drink has cayenne pepper for bringing your body temperature up, which makes your body work to get it cool again.

During this process, the body must burn a higher number of calories as it cools down, helping you shed some extra weight.

The Ingredients Needed:

To make this drink, use a glass of filtered water, one tablespoon of lemon juice, one tablespoon of organic, high-quality apple cider vinegar, half a teaspoon of cinnamon grounds and a pinch of cayenne.

You may also add stevia, quality maple syrup, or another natural sweetener. Don't use typical sugar. This should be stirred together and drank immediately.

Your Detoxing Cranberry Beverage:

Water and raw, healthy cranberry juice can help you clean out your kidneys, bowels, liver, and your lymphatic system of harmful, bad toxins.

Cranberries are full of compounds that draw fat out of your lymphatic system, since one of your lymphatic system's functions is absorbing fats from your digestion system, bringing them to your blood circulation.

For the cranberry juice you use, ensure that it's unsweetened, organic, and pure. Here are the ingredients for you detox beverage:

- One tablespoon of lemon juice.
- One tablespoon of apple cider vinegar.
- Half a cup of organic cranberry juice.
- Some water.

Mix the ingredients with as much water as you want until it tastes the way you prefer. You may make it strong or weak and flavor it with pure honey.

Your Weight Loss Green Tea Beverage:

Green tea helps you burn fat by boosting the metabolism. The mixture of honey, apple cider vinegar, and green tea combine to create a weight management drink that will also help you suppress your appetite.

Keep in mind that mixtures such as this work much better when combined with healthy eating habits and plenty of exercises. Before adding the apple cider vinegar to your tea, ensure that it's cooled enough and is no longer boiling, or it will ruin the apple cider vinegar's active culture.

Here are the ingredients you need to create this wonderful beverage:

- One tablespoon of apple cider vinegar.
- A single cup of organic green tea.

- Honey, if you prefer.

Make a cup of green tea, add some honey, then allow the tea to cool down. Add the apple cider vinegar to the mix. You can drink this right away to receive the benefits.

Vinegar Drizzle to cure your Sore Throat and Aid Digestion:

If you have issues like acid reflux (which can happen from not having enough acid in the stomach), ulcers, or colitis, apple cider vinegar mixed with some fermented vegetables can ease many different stomach issues.

The gentle acid present in fermentation is known as lactic acid, not acetic acid and can help to balance and heal the gut microbiome. Studies done on animals have shown that apple cider vinegar helps with digestion.

One study showed that apple cider vinegar could help ulcerative colitis by helping overall digestion issues. The study discovered that adding acetic acid to water helped bring better bacteria levels to the mice's guts.

In order to help your overall gut health, just make a concoction that consists of two tablespoons of apple cider vinegar, a glass of warm water, and a small amount of organic, raw honey.

Apple cider vinegar with ginger and honey for throat soreness is also effective and highly popular. You can also use this mix to help your sore throat, which comes recommended by a nurse from Pittsburgh University, Bonnie K. McMillen.

- Two tablespoons of pure water.

- One tablespoon of apple cider vinegar.

- A quarter teaspoon of powdered ginger.

- One tablespoon of organic, raw honey.

- A quarter teaspoon of cayenne pepper (optional).

To get the best results from this recipe, just take small sips once every two or three hours, swallowing it very slowly, so it has plenty of contact with your sore throat. Instead of directly sipping apple cider vinegar, dilute it with water.

A Vegetable Drizzle:

A yummy and simple recipe to put over salad greens, asparagus, or broccoli is a tablespoon of lemon juice, a tablespoon of apple cider vinegar, half a tablespoon of fresh, minced garlic, a bit of basil, and some black pepper.

If, after using apple cider vinegar for a while, you still don't like the taste, there are a few other creative ways you can ingest the liquid. Let's look at them now.

A delicious Cranberry Cocktail:

To make this tasty beverage, just mix together the following ingredients:

- Two tablespoons of organic cranberry juice.

- Half a cup of water.

- Two tablespoons of apple cider vinegar.

- Two tablespoons of organic maple syrup.

Mix all of these ingredients together in a glass and drink it immediately. Cranberries are a great addition since they are full of antioxidants, help heart health, aid digestion, and help to heal urinary tract infections.

Sweet, Mineral-rich Blaster Beverage:

This drink is not only sweet and tasty, but it's highly effective to help clean your body out. Here are the ingredients you will need to make it:

- Two tablespoons of molasses (black strap).

- Two tablespoons of apple cider vinegar.

- Two cups of water.

Blend these ingredients together and drink them right away. For the best results, you should take this first thing in the morning after waking up. It will deliver the great health advantages of apple cider vinegar while also bringing your body more calcium, manganese, magnesium, and iron from the molasses.

A Tomato Juice Lover's Drink:

This one won't be the favorite taste of most apple cider vinegar drinkers, but if you enjoy tomato juice, you will probably like it very much. Here are the ingredients you need to make it:

- Two teaspoons of fresh sea salt.
- Two tablespoons of organic apple cider vinegar.
- Canned or fresh tomato juice (as much as you want).
- Some hot sauce (if you prefer that).

This can be mixed together and drank immediately between meals.

Super Tangy Pink Juice:

To make the next item on our list, just gather and combine the following substances:

- Two tablespoons of organic, raw honey.
- Two tablespoons of apple cider vinegar.
- 1.5 cups of organic, fresh grapefruit (pink).

Blend all of this together in a glass and drink it down. You can use this before each meal during the day. If you want to lose some weight, this is very helpful. In addition, grapefruit can help you lower cholesterol while preventing arthritis and some forms of cancer.

A Simple Apple Cider Vinegar Shot:

For those who prefer a simpler method instead of an elaborate concoction, this shot may be perfect. Just mix together these ingredients to get the benefits of apple cider vinegar directly:

- A single tablespoon of apple juice or water.
- One tablespoon of organic apple cider vinegar.

Blend these two together and drink it back right away. You can hold your breath or plug your nose if you don't like the taste.

Increase the Brightness of your Chili:

Next time you're cooking chili at home, you can use apple cider vinegar as a way to increase flavor and brightness.

Apple cider vinegar can not only be used as a mouth rinse or whitener but may be used to clean your dentures or toothbrush. Just soak the brush in half a cup of water with a couple tablespoons of apple cider vinegar, then a tablespoon of pure baking soda.

Again, keep in mind that this acidity may cause tooth erosion, as proved in a single study. Another way to use apple cider vinegar is to kill your weeds, particularly the pesky ones growing on your sidewalk or driveway. Weed killers full of chemicals may harm your water system.

Natural Cures with Apple Cider Vinegar:

Apple cider vinegar is useful for may different conditions and can also be used as a strong cure and alternative to sometimes harmful traditional medical treatments.

As mentioned, you may use it to clean your house, your toothbrush, to kill weeds, and more! In addition, health professionals use it to target ailments and enhance changes in your lifestyle. Odds are, the liquid may enhance at least one area of your life. Here is a list of ways to use apple cider vinegar.

- **A Possible Remedy for Hair Loss:** We mentioned earlier that apple cider vinegar could help your hair become shinier and cure dandruff, but did you know that it can also be used as a remedy for hair loss?

- Simply add some apple cider vinegar to your hair, diluted with water, after you give it a regular shampoo and enjoy these benefits! Make sure you rinse well to get the smell out or use essential oils to make it less harsh.

- **A Strep Throat Remedy;** Most of us have had this common issue at least once in our life, but the powers of apple cider vinegar are very effective for treating it.

- Just mix some apple cider vinegar with warm water in a glass and gargle it a few times per day. How much you need depends on whether you're used to the liquid, but between one and three tablespoons should be sufficient.

- **Aiding Sinus Issues and Infections:** Traditionally, apple cider vinegar has been used to help treat sinus infections. To help your sinus infection disappear, just dilute a few tablespoons of apple cider vinegar in a glass of warm water.

- You may also mix some organic honey into it to make the taste nicer. This could cause your infection to be healed within just three days or so.

- **Healing Congestion Issues:** Apple cider vinegar has plenty of potassium, as we've mentioned, and this nutrient can help your body's mucus production decrease over time.

- In addition, apple cider vinegar has acetic acid that can help kill the growth of bacteria, including the bacteria responsible for nasal congestion issues. Drink some a couple times each day right before going to sleep diluted in water and mixed with organic honey.

- **Minimize your Pores:** In order to keep your pores looking nicer and smaller, just dab apple cider vinegar onto your face, diluted in water. You may also mix some baking soda in. Be sure to follow up with a quality, natural moisturizer.

- **Minimize Stretch Marks:** In order to make your stretch marks fade, just mix some apple cider vinegar with two parts warm water, blended with some raw honey. Put this in your stretch marks, leaving it to sit for two minutes before rinsing it off.

- Don't expect this to completely diminish your stretch marks, but it can help a lot with making them less noticeable.

- **Foot Fungus:** Along with curing foot odor, apple cider vinegar can help heal athlete's foot and other foot fungus problems. Just let your feet soak in a mix of warm water and vinegar, but don't pat dry after. Instead, let it dry on its own.

- **Curing the Hiccups:** One study showed that a teenager with a chronic hiccup issue solved the problem by mixing sugar and apple cider vinegar. Hiccups are the result of eating too much food, digesting sugary, fatty foods, or a low level of acid in the stomach.

- You can use apple cider vinegar to cure these, since it restores your stomach's balance of acid, easing the diaphragm spasms, and also triggering mouth and throat nerves, which contribute to the hiccups.

- **Helping Ear Infections:** As mentioned before, apple cider vinegar is a quality disinfectant. You may mix together water and rubbing alcohol, putting it into your ears with a dropper. Many people use this as a home remedy since it acts very fast compared to other methods.

- **Curing the Cold:** Apple cider vinegar works to boost your immune system, both protecting and strengthening your body when you get the cold or a flu.

Of course, many other home remedies with apple cider vinegar exist than just these ones, but it's a good start! It's a great remedy to use at home since it's cheap, easy to make, and very natural.

Here are some other Ailments that ACV can Help with:

- Menstrual cramps.
- Diabetes problems.
- A cough.
- Cleaning your wounds.
- Soothing mosquito bites.
- Bee stings.
- General inflammation and itching.
- Body detox.

Recommended Apple Cider Vinegar Brands

Apple cider vinegar on a regular basis can help you feel healthier and more energetic. You will be able to more effectively digest your food, feeling way lighter after eating.

You must also do conscious exercise and eating choices to get the full benefits. For years now, people have been reporting their amazing results from using this common, natural health remedy.

For many centuries, this vinegar has been put to use as a magical health tonic, curing high cholesterol, weak immune systems, heart issues, skin problems, diabetes, high blood pressure, and much more.

It can also be used to make your skin more youthful, to help combat hair loss, and to help you lose weight. Studies show that drinking this liquid each day can help you keep your blood sugar under control.

More Purported Apple Cider Vinegar Benefits:

- Treating varicose veins.
- Lowering blood pressure issues.
- Reducing cholesterol.
- Keeping osteoporosis away.
- Curing Psoriasis.
- Removing muscle stiffness.

- Soothing tired muscles.

- Strengthening your teeth and bones.

- Anti-aging effects on the skin.

- Helping to nourish your plants.

- Making your hair shinier and longer.

- Building up your immunity.

The Right Apple Cider Vinegar to Purchase:

Apple cider vinegar shouldn't be confused for white vinegar, which is found in the majority of home kitchens. Although, as mentioned before, all vinegar is pretty healthy, white vinegar is more useful for cooking, washing, and cleaning the house.

However, this vinegar has usually been refined, and therefore, doesn't have as many health advantages as pure, organic apple cider vinegar.

More about Apple Cider Vinegar:

Apple cider vinegar is made from a mix of crushed apple parts, also called apple must. This results from crushing entire apply, along with the seeds, stem, and skin.

The apple is brought through fermentation and oxygenation, converting the apple sugar into alcohol first. As it oxygenates, the present alcohol is changed into acetic acid, leading to the health values we've been discussing in this book.

Of course, the value is only retained when the vinegar is made the right way and is sold with the mother. So what is important to search for when purchasing apple cider vinegar?

Buy Organic:

Although this isn't an absolute must, it's best to buy your apple cider vinegar from organic apples, which will have natural sugar and no pesticides. In addition, the businesses that utilize organic apples probably take the care to follow a quality process for creating their apple cider vinegar.

Buy Unfiltered:

Buying unfiltered apple cider vinegar will help you make sure that it has the mother still in it, which is the muddy, grainy substance at the bottle's bottom. When you shake this up, the mother will float. The mother is the foundational essence of all apple cider vinegar, which stores the enzymes and provides all of the benefits you desire.

Buy Unpasteurized:

Always buy apple cider vinegar that is not pasteurized. The pasteurization process heats the liquid and kills of bad forms of bacteria, but unfortunately, this also gets rid of the bacteria you want.

Since you now know to search for unpasteurized, unfiltered, and organic apple cider vinegar, what brands should you look for? When it comes to choosing the right brand, keep in mind that more expensive doesn't always mean better. Actually, more affordable brands often give better value for what you pay.

The Best Apple Cider Vinegar Brands:

Here are some of the best apple cider vinegar which also offer you affordability:

Bragg Apple Cider Vinegar:

Bragg is among the absolute oldest of apple cider vinegar brands available today. Bragg is also very trusted in terms of vinegar brands. The company is based in California and uses apples that are native to the U.S.A. Due to this, they can control the quality of the apples they use.

Only organic apples are used, meaning that they don't have any pesticides or arsenic in them. In addition, Bragg uses wooden barrels to boost the fermentation process.

Bragg was founded by a man named Paul C. Bragg who advised some Olympian athletes, and his brand is backed up by his nutritionist daughter, Patricia Bragg.

Vitacost Apple Cider Vinegar:

Although Bragg is well-known for its range of apple cider vinegar, the brand Vitacost sells other health products, in addition, with the vinegar only being one purchase choice. Actually, Vitacost is more preferred than Dynamic Health and Bragg apple cider vinegar brands.

Vitacost says that the apple cider vinegar they make is the result of fermenting freshly pressed apples that are completely organic. The apple cider vinegar is not pasteurized, meaning it still has the mother. It has no sugar added, no colors added, and no artificial flavorings. In addition, it's suitable for vegetarians along with being kosher. For those seeking a quality, cheap brand, Vitacost is a great option.

Fleischmann's Apple Cider Vinegar:

You may also purchase apple cider vinegar from Fleischman's. This brand is based in California and has been creating vinegar since back in the 1920s. The brand started out using alcohol from the growth of baker's yeast.

As technology has advanced, baker's yeast lowered the alcohol production, causing the brand to enter into the specialty of creating just vinegar.

Dynamic Health and Apple Cider Vinegar:

Dynamic Health was created in 1994 and has been providing products and health supplements that are halal-certified, fully organic, and also available in both capsule and liquid forms.

The apple cider vinegar products from Dynamic Health are very competitive, offering quality value for what you spend.

To Summarize:

To summarize, each of these brands covered are great. The companies use organic, fresh-pressed apples that create unpasteurized, unfiltered, raw, organic apple cider vinegar. Each of these still has the healthful mother intact.

You don't have to store your purchased apple cider vinegar in the fridge, but you should avoid sunlight and keep it in glass rather than plastic.

Where to Buy Apple Cider Vinegar:

Apple cider vinegar can be made on your own, as we covered earlier in the book, but you can usually find it at health food stores, online, or even at ordinary grocery stores. In order to find a quality brand, you will probably have a better look at a specialty health store.

CHAPTER 5

PRECAUTIONS AND RECOMMENDATIONS

Apple cider vinegar not only has amazing health benefits but is completely safe to ingest. However, if you aren't careful, some side effects could occur. Do the side effects from apple cider vinegar mean that it isn't safe to ingest? Let's look at the details of this question.

Let's first be clear on one thing; apple cider vinegar is very safe to ingest. A wonderful supplement for great health, the benefits of apple cider vinegar are very numerous.

From utilizing it to tone your skin to making your hair nicer, and also to help you lose weight, you shouldn't miss out on apple cider vinegar. So why is there some concern about how safe consuming apple cider vinegar is, along with possible side effects?

There's a simple answer to that question. Apple cider vinegar is acidic, so consider the following before committing to a daily supplement of it.

What Amount is Safe to Consume?

Consuming too much apple cider vinegar can hinder your body from effectively and fully absorbing calcium. For this reason, don't take over 30 ml per day.

When should it be Ingested?

As stated and shown, apple cider vinegar has many benefits, but it's best to consult a doctor if you have any concerns or questions about whether it's right for you.

This is especially important if you want to use it to cure stomach ailments, kidney problems, wart removal, liver detox, sore throat problems, or to control your blood sugar.

When shouldn't you use ACV?

Although drinking apple cider vinegar in a safe, recommended amount, in some cases, there isn't a lot of information freely available on how safe it is to consume apple cider vinegar.

If a woman is breastfeeding or pregnant, she shouldn't consume too much apple cider vinegar unless her doctor specifically suggests or approves it. In addition, if you have a disease of any kind, please consult your doctor before you ingest this liquid to prevent any side effects from occurring.

Now that you are aware of some of the side effects that may come from apple cider vinegar, you should know more about it before drinking it regularly.

Some of the Possible Side Effects of Apple Cider Vinegar:

Low Levels of Potassium:

Since apple cider vinegar is so acidic, one common issue with ingesting too much of it is lowered levels of potassium in your blood. If you have been drinking apple cider vinegar and notice low blood pressure, cramps, or nausea, please ask your doctor to look into the reasons behind this. It may be due to consuming too much apple cider vinegar.

Irritation of the Throat:

As mentioned earlier in the book, apple cider vinegar can bring relief to throat soreness, but consuming it too much could lead to the opposite effect, irritating your throat and worsening the condition.

Lowered Density in the Bones:

Excessive use or over-dosage of this liquid could lead to lowered bone density in your body. It could make your bones weaker, indirectly increasing the risk of breaking your bones from a hard fall or minor accident.

Erosion of Tooth Enamel:

We already briefly discussed the risk of your tooth enamel being eroded from too much apple cider vinegar. Even soda heightens the risk of tooth erosion because of the drink's acetic makeup.

In a similar way, apple cider vinegar being used often isn't very different and can lead to both decay and the general erosion of your teeth.

Causing Skin Irritation:

If you use apple cider vinegar for your skin, particularly on the sensitive skin of your face, be careful. If you have sensitive skin, it's best to first consult an expert. As said before, always dilute this liquid before you apply it to your face reducing the risk of skin burn or irritation.

Taking Precautions before Use of ACV:

- Make sure you avoid using ACV without dilution unless a health expert or doctor has specifically guided you to do so.

- Don't ever consume apple cider vinegar more than the safe, recommended amounts or it could cause your body harm.

- In order to gain the full possible health benefits of apple cider vinegar, it's best to ask your doctor how much he or she recommends that you take. This way, you will stay safe and reduce risks of health problems.

- Keep in mind that apple cider vinegar is very safe for your body as long as you follow these guidelines for safe consumption.

Once you observe all of the rules above, you should be fine to drink apple cider vinegar every day.

CHAPTER 6

BONUS: APPLE CIDER VINEGAR IN TREATMENT OF CELLULITE

Cellulite is an embarrassing problem that affects many people, mostly women. Cellulite consists of fat cells under the skin that are free floating. The appearance of cellulite is very distinct and appears like cottage cheese or a dimpled orange peel surface. Genetics, hormones, and a lack of healthy habits are the main causes of this problem.

You have to get rid of it right away when it shows up because cellulite usually worsens as you age. There are a few different effective methods that can pause or slow down this occurrence, minimizing the look of cellulite on your body, especially on the thighs.

Apple cider vinegar is one effective method for doing that. We will discuss how and then give some other natural remedies for curing cellulite. For the best results, use these in combination.

How does Apple Cider Vinegar helps with Cellulite?

Apple cider vinegar contains strong astringent properties, along with its previously mentioned skin-toning abilities that will help your body get rid of cellulite, the freely floating cells of fat just below your skin.

There are several components present in apple cider vinegar that can help water retention and with flushing out toxins near your stomach and thighs, which goes a long way to reducing the unattractive look of cellulite. Along with this, apple cider vinegar aids in weight loss, improving your skin's elasticity.

Your Home Cellulite-Busting ACV Recipe:

In order to reap the benefits from this wonderful liquid to fight your cellulite, just follow these very simple instructions:

- Mix three parts apple cider vinegar with one-part coconut or olive oil, then place this in the area that is affected.

- Massage the mixture into your skin for 15 to 20 minutes. This can be repeated two times per day until you see an improvement.

- You may also mix two tablespoons of unfiltered, raw apple cider vinegar with a teaspoon of organic, raw honey in a warm glass of filtered water. This can be drunk twice per day, every day.

This drink will help your body fight imbalances in your hormones, which can lead to a weight gain issue.

How Does ACV Help Remove Cellulite?

Apple cider vinegar helps your body get rid of this problem because of the calcium, magnesium, and potassium present within it. Each of these elements contributes to flushing toxins out of your body, along with reducing water retention in both the stomach and the thighs.

This process helps to reduce cellulite and general body bloating, helping you shed extra pounds. Lower amounts of fat on the body means lower pockets of cellulite on the body.

Here is a useful recipe for helping to reduce cellulite, which can be used in conjunction with the one above:

- Combine two parts warm water with one-part ACV. You can optionally add raw honey, too.

- Spread this mixture over your affected body areas and allow it to sit for a half hour. It can then be rinsed off using lukewarm water.

- Do this twice a day to reach your desired result.

- On the other hand, you can mix water with apple cider vinegar in two equal amounts, rubbing it over your thighs or other areas of cellulite.

- This body part should be wrapped up in Saran wrap, then rinsed off with water. This can be done once per day until your cellulite goes away.

Note that you may also add a teaspoon of raw honey to two tablespoons of ACV, drinking this twice a day, every day.

Other Natural Remedies for Cellulite to use with ACV:

Apple cider vinegar isn't the only useful ingredient for helping you fight cellulite. You may use the following remedies to make the apple cider vinegar treatment even more effective.

Using Coffee Grounds to Fight Cellulite:

You can use coffee grounds to make an exfoliating body scrub. This will take away old, dead cells of the skin, generate healthier, newer cells. In addition, drinking coffee often can help improve your body's blood circulation. Just follow these steps to gain the wonderful cellulite-blasting properties from coffee:

- Combine olive oil or liquid coconut oil (two tablespoons) with three tablespoons of raw sugar and a quarter cup of coarse coffee grounds (fresh or used). Once this paste is blended, it can be spread over the affected area.

- Allow this to sit for a few minutes after you apply it with firm pressure, then rinse the mixture off your skin with warm (not hot) water.

- This solution can be used up to three times each week to get the results you desire. Keep in mind that you can store any leftover materials in a jar to use later.

- In addition, you may create an olive oil and coffee warp. Just heat up a bit of virgin olive oil with half a cup of coarse coffee grounds in your microwave. Don't heat them for over 20 seconds or it will get too hot.

- This mixture should be spread over your cellulite, then covered up with Saran wrap. Allow it to sit for a half hour before rinsing it from your body. This can be done twice weekly until your cellulite improves.

Using Juniper Oil to Heal Cellulite:

Juniper oil contains many valuable detoxifying ingredients, helping to fight fluid retention, which in turn can treat cellulite in your body. To make use of this amazing oil, just follow these steps:

- Combine 15 drops of this oil in a quarter cup of melted coconut oil or organic olive oil.

- Spread this oil over your cellulite and let it sit for 15 minutes each time you use the treatment.

- This can be done two times each day. Once 30 days have passed, your skin in that area will appear firmer and softer to the touch.

Using Seaweed to Fight Cellulite:

Seaweed is a useful and natural agent of exfoliation for the skin. It helps your body stimulate blood circulation, flushes out toxins, and improves the texture of your skin. All of this combines to help reduce the look of your cellulite. Just follow these steps to benefit from seaweed for fighting cellulite:

- Combine a few tablespoons of seaweed (make sure it's ground) with a quarter cup of extra virgin olive oil and a quarter cup of pure sea salt. This can be found in most health stores in America.

- You may mix some of your favorite essential oils into this mix to make it smell nice, then rub it onto your cellulite, leaving it to sit for 15 minutes and then rinsing it off in a warm shower.

- Once this has been applied and you have rinsed it off, make sure you use a moisturizer to heighten the effects.

- This natural remedy can be utilized every day for weeks at a time, and the extra mixture may be stored away in an airtight container to use later on.

- In addition, you may bathe with some seaweed in the water, which can help you reduce cellulite on your body. To do this just add a few sheets of seaweed into your tub, then fill it with warm or hot water.

- Soak in your tub for at least a half hour and perform this two times a day to get the highest number of benefits.

Cellulite can be a really embarrassing problem, leading you to want to hide your body and avoid swimsuits. You shouldn't have to live with this anymore, and with these natural recipes, you have a way to naturally change that.

Using some of these suggested natural remedies you now have the potential to remove cellulite within just a month: combined with a healthy diet, lifestyle and moderate exercise routine.

..And don't forget to use apple cider vinegar for all of the other amazing benefits we've covered throughout this book. Good luck!

CONCLUSION

Thank you for reading *Apple Cider Vinegar: Natural Weight Loss, Glowing Health and Skin, Natural Cures, and Alkaline Healing with Apple Cider Vinegar.*

Taking Action For Your Health:

Hopefully, this book has shown you some of the many ways that you can start to use the wonderful apple cider vinegar to improve your health and improve your life overall. Making this miracle liquid at home is very simple and easy, and that way, you can be sure it's organic and raw

Whether you want a chemical-free method for cleaning your kitchen, wish to help cure your acne, or want to lose some weight, apple cider vinegar can help!

Finally, if you found this book enlightening and useful, please take the time to leave it a positive review on Amazon. Thank you and good luck!

Made in the USA
Middletown, DE
07 March 2019